D0859911

Joy Is a

Plum Colored

Acrobat

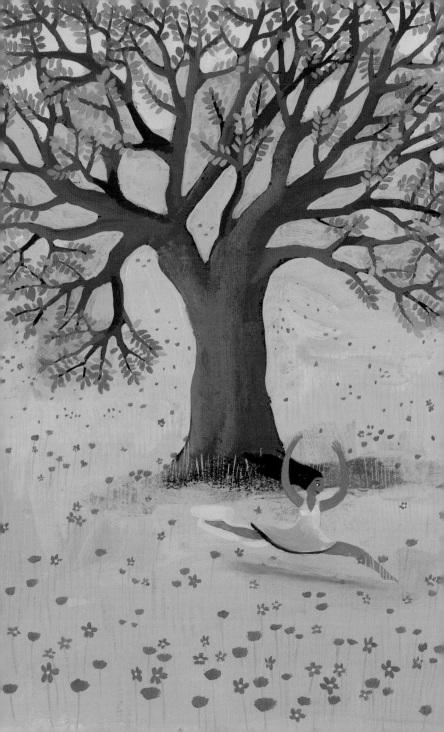

Joy Is a
Plum Colored
Acrobat

45
Life-Affirming
Visualizations for
Breast Cancer
Treatment and
Recovery

Wendy Burton

Illustrations by Simona Mulazzani

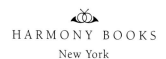

HARMONY BOOKS

New York

Published by Harmony Books, New York, New York. Member of the Crown
Publishing Group, a division of Random House, Inc.
www.crownpublishing.com

HARMONY BOOKS is a registered trademark and the Harmony Books colophon
is a trademark of Random House, Inc.

Printed in China

Design by Wendy Burton / For A Small Fee, Inc.

Library of Congress Cataloging-in-Publication Data

Burton, Wendy, 1951
  Joy is a plum-colored acrobat : 45 life-affirming
visualizations for breast cancer treatment and recovery /
Wendy Burton ; illustrations by Simona Mulazzani—1st
ed.
Includes bibliographical references.
  (Hardcover)
1. Breast—Cancer—Treatment. 2. Visualization.
3. Imagery (Psychology) I. Title.
  RC280.B8B845 2004
  616.99´44906—dc22
  2003026118

ISBN 1-4000-5479-6

10 9 8 7 6 5 4 3 2 1

First Edition

To my husband, Jeff, who cradles me in love.

To Dr. Emily Sonnenblick, Dr. Alexander Swistel,

Pat Burbridge, and Rob Wallin:

All of you are my heroes.

Contents

Introduction

IT IS A MYSTERY TO ME why I was able to find at the core of my experience with cancer a deep sense of joy and gratitude. Inexplicably I felt I was in a state of grace. Our instincts rightly tell us that cancer is darkly frightening. It is life-threatening. But when it showed up, unbidden and unwelcome at my doorstep, I was somehow able to take a few very deep breaths and embrace this stranger. It wasn't that my arms were open to the *cancer*. It was more about being open to the journey that the diagnosis of cancer would take me on. I didn't feel as if I had chosen this ride, but since I was on it, I wanted to be on it with clarity and an open heart.

Perhaps it is significant that my diagnosis was a relatively easy one. DCIS (ductal carcinoma in situ) is a very treatable form of breast cancer, and mine was detected early. A more difficult diagnosis would have been a far greater challenge for me.

I was also fortunate enough to have had role models who helped me maintain a certain lightness of heart and spirit. I had watched my mother face cancer with dignity and grace and my brother face it with glowing inner strength and serenity. And then I was given some tools.

A social worker at the Dyson Cancer Center at the Vassar

Brothers Medical Center in Poughkeepsie, New York, passed along a meditation tape made by Belleruth Naparstek called *Relaxation and Guided Imagery for Patients Undergoing Radiation Therapy*. It taught me to relax as completely as possible, and then respond to guided imagery as my own imagination saw fit. At first I listened to the tape every day, and followed Belleruth's script closely. Then one day I simply took off on my own.

Joy became the central theme of my voyage through cancer. By relaxing deeply and letting my imagination lead the way, I created vibrant, energetic, whimsical images to brighten the experiences I was having, like the colorized version of *The Wizard of Oz*. These images made me happy. They strengthened and delighted me.

Who gave me the Technicolor glasses that I have worn throughout my treatment? I don't know. But my life changed profoundly the moment that the tiny Cirque du Soleil acrobats showed up in my imagination to help me usher out my unwanted cancer cells with their brilliant energy and pizzazz. I had no use for the warrior imagery that so many people automatically thrust at me when they heard I had cancer. *Kill the cancer! Annihilate those horrible cells! You are such a warrior!* None of those images worked for me. I just felt so much love for my body—for letting me know in the form of minuscule microcalcifications that something was amiss. How wise of it to do that! I realized I wanted to celebrate my body, and equip it with lively, lovely, colorful helpers to accompany me on the way to wellness. They could take care of the cancer just as well as an arsenal of Uzis. After my acrobats showed up, I found that if I simply took visual dictation from my imagination, it would lead me on fantastic journeys that were infused with the simple gift of joy.

The visualizations I have done during the course of my treatment for cancer served as a wonderful lens through which to filter my experience. My hope is that whatever stage your cancer is in, visualizations may ease your way as they did mine, and help you to heal—through surgery, radiation, or chemotherapy. I was able to lift myself out of what could have been a sterile medical experience, full of fear and uncertainty, into a fertile, creative, warm, and safe state of mind where I gave myself quite a bit of control over the situation I found myself in.

My other hope is that the images that have come to me over the course of my treatment might be helpful to you. They have given me a great deal of pleasure, insight, and comfort. They have guided me toward health. Perhaps they can be springboards for your own imagination. May your voyages bring you joy, comfort, and health.

FIVE WORDS OF ADVICE: JUST TRUST IN YOUR IMAGINATION! Give it free rein to take you wherever it has the inclination to go. When we relax deeply enough, and stop trying to control the course of these journeys, our subconscious seems to be able to provide just what we need at the moment we need it. When I first started to do these visualizations I would think I knew in advance where I was going. *I'm off to Third Mesa again. Time for another visit with that Hopi medicine woman!* But then I might close my eyes, clear my head and realize I was boarding a spaceship with a humongous fan mounted on the nosecone. *Guess I'm not going to Third Mesa today* was a response that yielded better results than *Get off that spaceship and go to the desert.* So my advice is to trust in your imagination, put on your seatbelt, and *let 'er rip!*

WHY VISUALIZATIONS?

DREAMS ARE THE INTERMEDIARIES between our conscious and unconscious minds. Sometimes direct, often cloaked in symbolism and even humor, the visual language of dreams is, of course, innate to all of us. This is the language with which the subconscious speaks. It makes perfect sense that we can harness that imagery—pulling it up from deep within us or sending it back to our deeper minds in a directed way—in order to help ourselves heal.

Research has been done in hospitals around the country confirming the impact that directed imagery, or visualizations, can have on a patient's health. Visualizations have been used to lower blood pressure, increase the number of white blood cells in the bloodstream, reduce pain, lessen anxiety, and enable patients to mend more quickly.

There is an entire body of literature devoted to visualization and sports performance. *The Inner Game of Tennis,* written by W. Timothy Gallwey and published in 1974, was revolutionary in its time, showing how a tennis player could improve his or her performance drastically by working on the "inner" game. Now entire sections in bookstores are devoted to sports psychology, teaching athletes how to maximize the mind/body connection for optimum performance. Often when we see an athlete deeply focused before she acts, she is visualizing the outcome—whether it's a perfect routine on the balance beam or a flawless triple jackknife off the diving board. We use visualizations to "see" ourselves succeed.

Visualizations can help our bodies to mobilize white blood cells or to protect healthy cells during treatment. We *can* communicate with our bodies. We are psychobiological beings. Not only can we make ourselves feel better emotionally, which is no small accomplishment, we can help ourselves to heal.

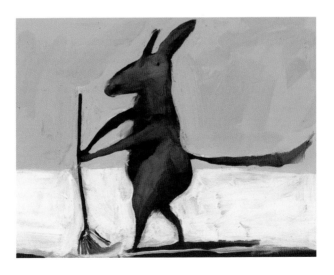

How to Prepare Yourself to Visualize

I suggest that you go to a favorite room, a place where you find sanctuary. Begin by making yourself comfortable, either reclining on a bed, resting on a well-worn couch, or sitting in a favorite easy chair. I like to retreat to the quiet, peaceful refuge of my bedroom. I prop myself up with pillows behind my back, arms resting gently by my sides. My legs are uncrossed, and sometimes I put an extra pillow underneath my knees. I try to make sure that the house will be quiet for twenty minutes or so.

Try to create this time for yourself every day, if you can. For one thing, the rest itself will do you good. Treatment for breast cancer can cause fatigue, and a twenty-minute time-out every day is healing in and of itself. Just as important, doing visualizations every day becomes a practice, like daily meditation or sitting zazen. It provides a supportive structure to your day, and is a true present, wrapped up in brightly colored gift wrap, that you can give yourself.

Begin to relax by taking slow, deep, cleansing breaths. If you are aware of tension in your body, or anxiety camped out in tight places, try to direct your breath to those areas, one at a time. As you breathe out, try to usher that tension or anxiety out on the exhale. Take your time. This quiet space that you are carving out for yourself can provide a potent healing experience, and you deserve to feel unhurried. You are allowing yourself to go on a journey into your own interior, and if you can, imagine yourself standing with arms wide open in a favorite field, ready to embrace this experience. Trust that it will bring you exactly what it is that you currently need.

Continue to breathe quietly in and out. What I like to do, on an inhalation, is to close my eyes, gently rolling them backward, and imagine I'm looking into the open screening room of my mind. You can imagine a blank movie screen, or an amphitheater under the stars, but try to clear a space for your visualization to unfold. When I listen to guided imagery tapes, the speaker generally helps me select the setting for the journey I will take. When I'm visualizing on my own, I don't know in advance who will step into that amphitheater, or where that amphitheater might be. But, magically, the scenery appears and my helpmates show up. It might be my mom; it might be the acrobats I'm going to tell you about. I might be flying through the night air, or diving under turquoise water.

When I relax deeply enough, my subconscious always seems to know where it needs to take me. Just trust that yours will know too. Don't worry if the images don't come right away. Give yourself time, and permission to get used to the process. In the meantime, it might be useful to listen to a guided imagery tape just to get started. Or simply hitchhike along with me on the visualizations I am going to describe.

Author's note: I was taught a technique for self-hypnosis that enabled me to relax quite deeply. I believe this helped me considerably on my voyages into the "interior." There are professional clinical hypnotists who can teach you this skill and a large canon of work on visualization and relaxation techniques. I have listed a few of them in the bibliography. But to begin, I simply want to provide some easy and effective techniques to get you relaxed and on your way.

PRAYER FOR AN OPEN HEART

It goes without saying that nobody in their right mind wants to hear

"cancer" come out of their doctor's mouth. It is a frightening,

heart-stopping word. We think of lives cut short, of the struggles our

friends and family may have endured, of what it will mean to feel

we have lost control of our own destiny.

This visualization is about turning the angle of our mind a few

degrees away from fear and toward the direction of fully embracing

the challenge of what life has handed us at this particular moment.

It's about opening our arms and hearts to what we have been given

and to acceptance, so we can put on our seatbelts and wholeheartedly

go along for the ride, wherever it might take us. We don't need to be

victims. We can be explorers instead.

A WHEAT-COLORED FIELD

I am standing alone in an enormous wheat-colored field. It extends to the horizon in all four directions. All I can see is field and sky, the sky a softly lit pale blue. I am standing barefoot in the center of this field, with my legs planted firmly at shoulder width, and my arms stretched out wide in an embrace that takes in all that my eyes can see. I turn slowly in a circle and can feel the earth's energy come up through the soles of my feet. I feel the coolness of the air gently pass over my skin. I absorb these gifts of energy, these gentle reminders of the power and mysteries the earth offers, with gratitude. I take a deep, deep breath and I welcome the rite of passage I am about to embark upon. Like Amelia Earhart, I will strap on my aviator's cap and fly willingly into the unknown.

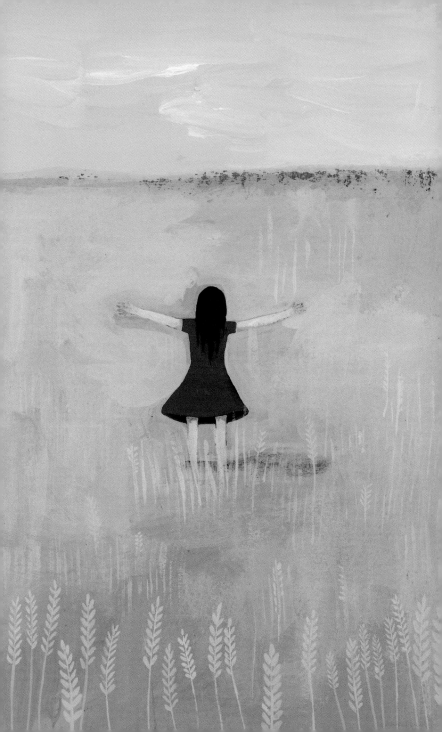

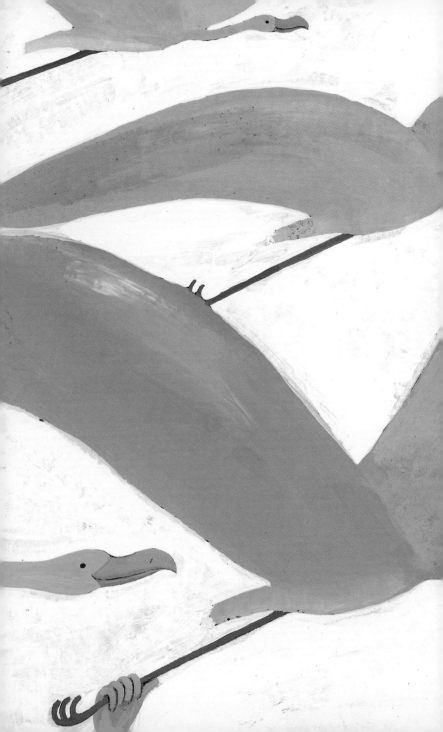

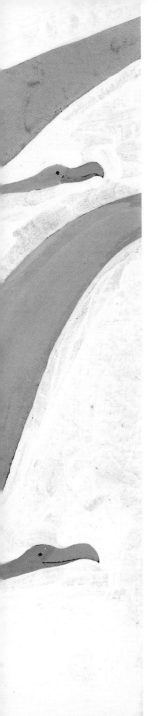

Visualizations *for* Protection: Radiation

The treatment of my breast under the linear accelerator involved exposing the healthy tissue to radiation as well as any cancer cells that might have been left behind after surgery. Healthy cells can regenerate after radiation. Cancer cells should not. Although the daily dose of radiation that I underwent literally happened in minutes, I still wanted to provide my healthy breast cells with some kind of special protection during treatment. So once I was positioned on the table, the technicians had left the room, and the linear accelerator had begun the whirring sound it made before treatment actually started, I closed my eyes, and this is what I imagined:

BEAUTIFULLY COLORED BEACH UMBRELLAS

I am handing them out to all of my healthy cells. These umbrellas are HUGE! They are orange and purple and ruby red, metallic gold, turquoise blue, and magenta. They all open magically with a loud snap the moment the radiant beam comes on. It is a glorious day at the beach—warm light shining down and all of these enormous umbrellas opening at the same time. *Only the cancer cells don't get any!* They come directly into contact with this strong, very focused, and intelligent light. And they start to melt away.

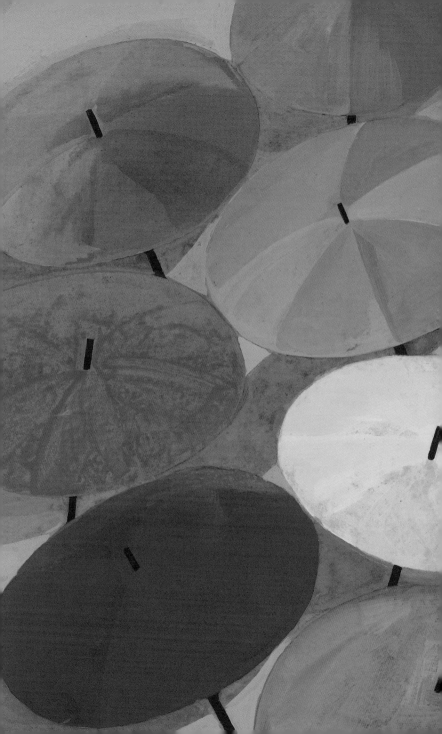

GIGANTIC PINK FLAMINGOS

When the whirring sound begins, I close my eyes, and an enormous flock of shocking pink flamingos appears. These are no ordinary flamingos—their wingspan is triple that of your garden-variety flamingo, casting a deep protective shadow across my breast. In addition, these large birds are made of starched silk—I wouldn't want to subject real flamingos to radiation. Each healthy cell holds on to an outstretched flamingo leg and is shielded from the light. My cancer cells are not visited by flamingos. They, instead, began to vaporize in the intensity of the beam.

MONARCH BUTTERFLIES

I once lived in Pacific Grove, California. At the same time each year, the town would be blanketed by what seemed like a billion monarch butterflies that were passing through on their annual migration. Everywhere you looked, you could see the orange and black beauties. In this visualization, as the whirring begins, my healthy cells are enveloped in a cloud of these gorgeous, iridescent butterflies. They themselves are somehow protected from the radiant light—and they are savvy enough to cover only my healthy tissue. The cancer cells look up and see nary a wing beating—just the incandescent light that will turn them into dust.

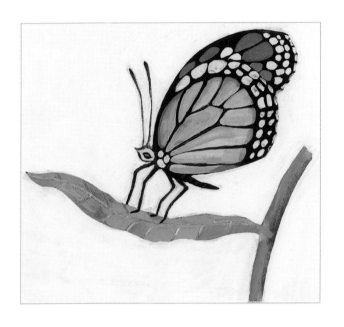

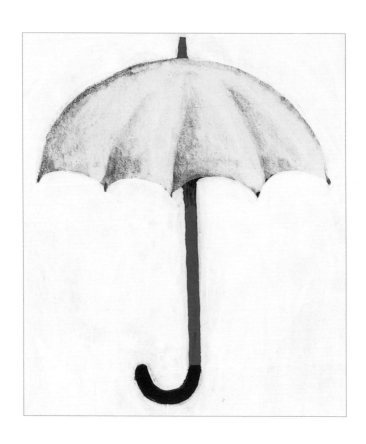

The three images I have just described gave me great comfort. The beach umbrellas in particular would snap open for me almost every single day, and I welcomed them. What I learned about my imagination was that it could still surprise me. The last two images sneaked up on me toward the end of treatment, and showed me that I was trying to tell myself something new.

THE WHITE UMBRELLAS

I was once again on the table, closing my eyes, breathing quietly—and this time when the umbrellas snapped open, *they were all white!* Where did all of my bright colors go? I was very surprised. I must have been telling myself that the radiation had truly worked. I believe my system was clear of cancer cells, and lily white was the blessing of the day.

INVISIBLE PROTECTIVE COATING

For my final treatment, something different happened. I was in my familiar position, arm up, eyes closed, when the machine came on to deliver its final dose. The moment was weighted with significance for me. Uh oh. No umbrellas popped open. Instead the beam seemed to be delivering a protective sealer to my healthy breast tissue. The cancer cells were gone, and I imagined a fine and clear spray of protection coating me and keeping me safe as I stepped off the treatment table and into my Life After Cancer.

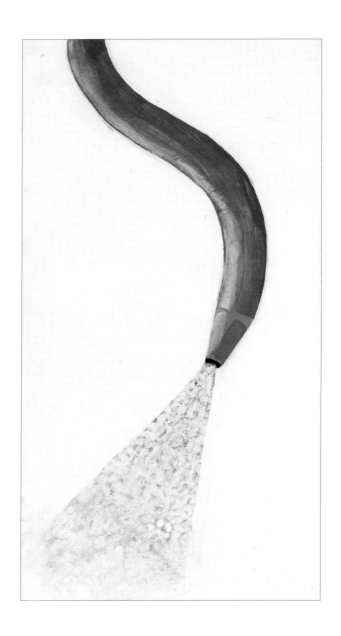

31

Visualizations *for* Protection: Chemotherapy

My particular course of treatment did not call for the use of chemotherapy, so I did not experience it firsthand. I have read about it, and I have spoken with many women who have undergone this form of treatment. I understand that it can be much more difficult than what I underwent, but I have tried hard to imagine what it might be like. I think about the intra-venous liquid as a delivery system for all kinds of wonderful helpers. Their vigilance and skills, be they miners or cowgirls at the rodeo, are mingled with the alchemical magic of the chemotherapy. The process of protecting healthy cells looked different to me when I visualized myself preparing for chemotherapy. This is what I saw:

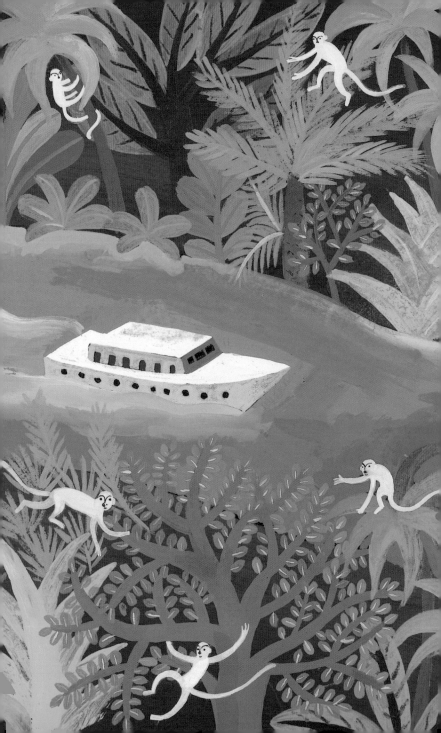

CRUISING DOWN THE AMAZON

I am sitting in a comfortable lounge chair, on board a pleasure boat that is cruising down the Amazon. We can see the rain forest on either side of the river. I close my eyes as the clear liquid that will deliver me back to health begins to drip down the tubing and into my body. In just an instant, all of my healthy cells have donned bright yellow rain slickers—pants and a hooded jacket. They are protected from harm by this resilient, impenetrable garb. My cancer cells are not outfitted with the rain gear, and they melt away as I sit watching little yellow squirrel monkeys jump from treetop to treetop as we meander peacefully down the river.

HONEY

I am lying back in a comfortable lounger, waiting for my treatment to begin. In my mind, while the nurse is needed elsewhere, I mix some golden honey in with the chemistry that will cure me. When the drip begins, the sweet, protective honey seeks out my healthy cells, and coats them entirely. They are left unharmed by the chemo. My cancer cells are left uncoated, and helplessly disintegrate.

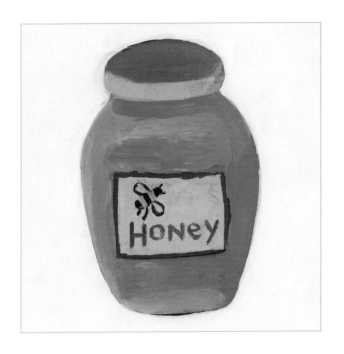

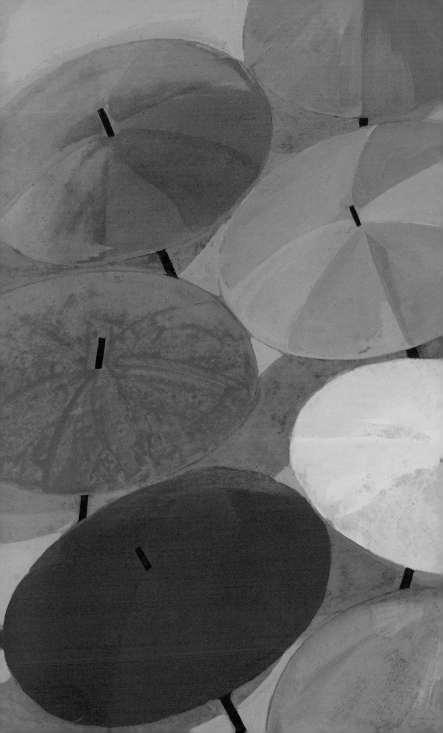

BEACH UMBRELLAS REDUX

It's raining inside my body! I am lying back in my
Barcalounger. The clear healing liquid is moving through the
tube, pouring down into my bloodstream. The moment the
drip begins, I hand out enormous, brightly colored umbrellas
to all of my healthy cells: orange and crimson, turquoise and
purple, magenta and gold. The healthy cells stay warm and
protected from the chemical rain. I do not hand out umbrellas
to my cancer cells. They get soaked, are rendered harmless,
and go metaphorically down the drain.

Visualizations
for Treatment:
Radiation

I felt so fortunate to be receiving radiation therapy. If I had known how to tap-dance, I would have tap-danced my way on to the treatment table every morning. So I pictured it instead. I was happy that there was something I could be doing to help cure myself. My enthusiasm might have seemed a little alarming to the technicians at first, but it was genuine. Bring those radiation beams on down and let me get started!

The radiation treatments lasted less than two minutes each day—not a whole lot of time to settle down and let my imagination wander. So at least once a day, usually in the afternoon, I would take twenty minutes or so and give myself the gift of imagination. I would retire to the sanctuary of our bedroom, get comfortable on the bed, relax deeply by breathing and clearing my mind, and either follow Belleruth's guided imagery tape or simply lie back and watch the movie that would magically appear on the blank movie screen in my mind.

The best instruction I can give is to try not to direct traffic. Our imaginations are rich, fertile places. They don't need to be microman-aged. Left to their own magic, they can take our breath away with their ingenuity and caprice. Because I lived in California for over a decade, the beauty of that state—a state that had offered me so many exquisite and varied environments to visit and explore—informs many of my images. Your experiences will most likely be different from mine. My field of lupine in Carmel Valley may be an apple orchard in upstate New York to you. Death Valley may become a cool pine forest deep in the White Mountains of New Hampshire. The High Sierra may instead be a windswept beach in the Bahamas. So again, please think about my visualizations loosely, as road maps that will take you to your own unique landscapes.

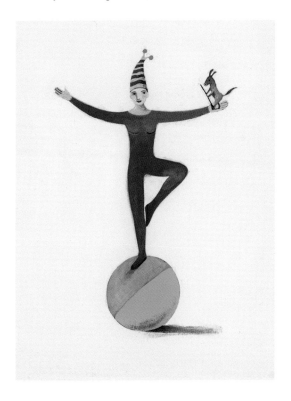

CIRQUE DU SOLEIL ACROBATS

These teeny-weeny acrobats have been my joyful companions almost every single day. I picture them inside my breast ducts, wearing their glorious, iridescent body suits, which cover them from the top of their head to their tiny acrobat toes. They are dressed in shiny sparkling material—purple and crimson, pumpkin and metallic gold, yellow and plum. They are twirling and turning somersaults, they are vaulting and springing high in the air doing backflips and pirouettes, all the while moving the cancer cells down through the tunnels of my breast ducts with their little feet and their flying bodies—down the ducts and magically out of me.

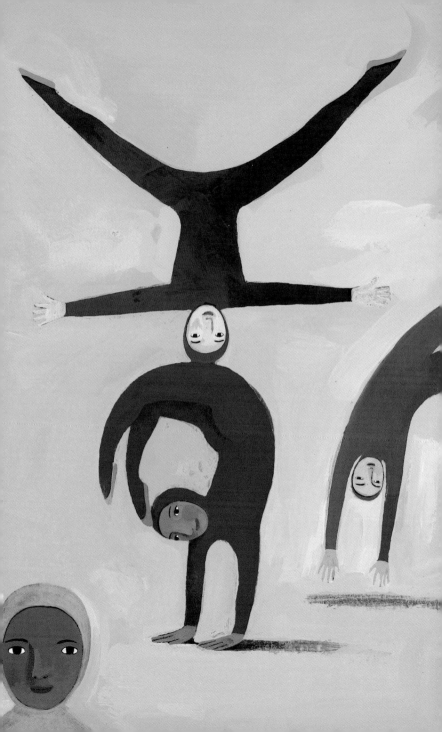

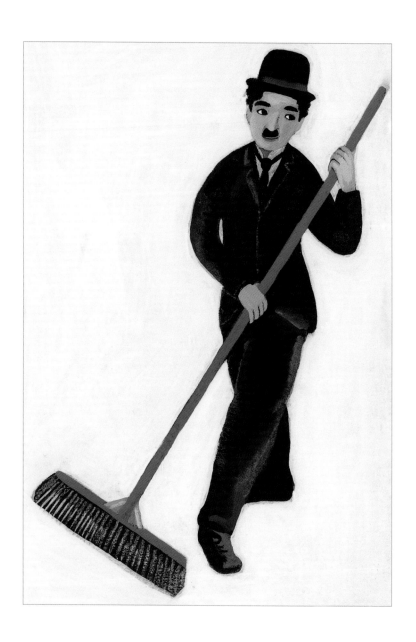

CHARLIE CHAPLIN

I picture Charlie Chaplin, only there are hundreds of him in my breast ducts. And they all have large industrial brooms. They waddle through my ducts in that stiff-legged signature walk, pushing their giant brooms in front of them, sweeping sweeping sweeping out the dried, discarded cancer cells. Occasionally they may stop in unison to tip their tiny bowler hats at me, but mainly they are very busy sweeping.

HULA DANCERS

I am in Kona, on the island of Hawaii. I am on a beach, warming my toes in the sand as the sun begins to set. There are a dozen hula dancers, with purple orchids around their necks, wearing grass skirts with bracelets around their ankles. They are dancing inside my breast. The swaying motion of the hula dancers' bodies mesmerizes my cancer cells. The dancers' arms undulate in one direction as their hips sway in the other. With each powerful rotation of their hips, they knock the hypnotized cancer cells out of my body and into the blue Pacific.

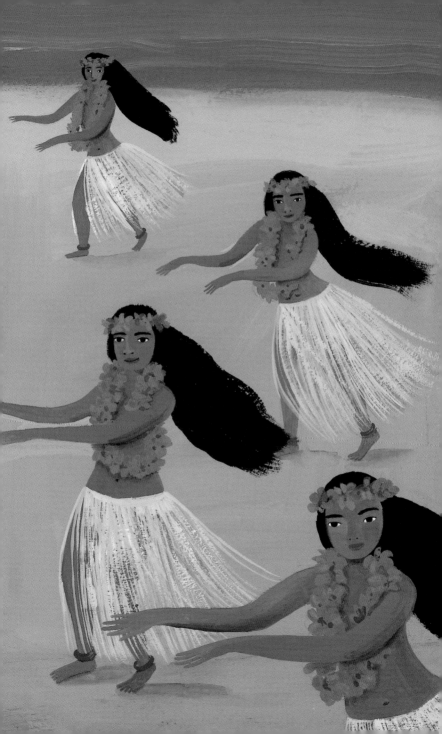

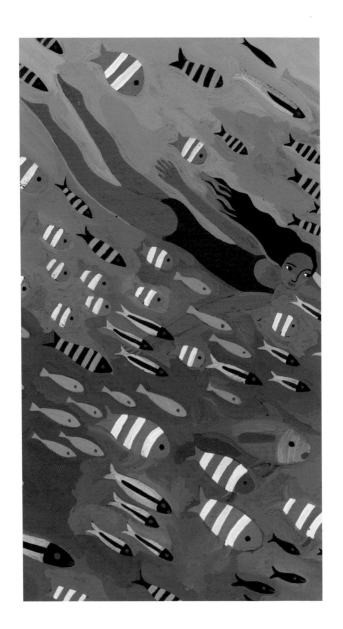

TROPICAL FISH

Sometimes I am underwater, but always I am able to breathe easily. I must have gills. I dive into the indigo water, and swim down and down and down, pulling myself deeper and deeper with strong arms. I bump up against dolphins and whales. Sometimes I even hitch a ride down, holding on to a dorsal fin or climbing on to a broad back. There are pint-sized tropical fish, yellow and black or turquoise and orange, swimming in schools all around me. I realize that those tiny fish are swimming inside me as well as around me—that they are in my breast ducts and with their fish noses gently pushing the cancer cells out. And maybe other little fish that are hungry see those cancer cells in the water and immediately eat them up—all part of the food chain.

WHEN THE SAINTS GO MARCHING IN

I am in New Orleans. It might be Mardi Gras. I'm not sure, but there is a huge parade in progress and it is going on inside of my breast ducts. As far as I can see, line after line of miniature trumpet and trombone players are high-stepping and playing "When the Saints Go Marching In." It is a riotous festival atmosphere, with miniature baton twirlers kicking high and twirling their silver batons overhead. The sound of the horns fills everything, and with each blast of the instruments, my desiccated cancer cells get hooted right out of my body, into the ozone and far away from me.

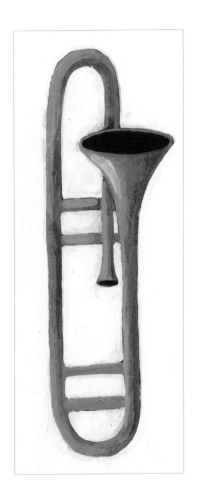

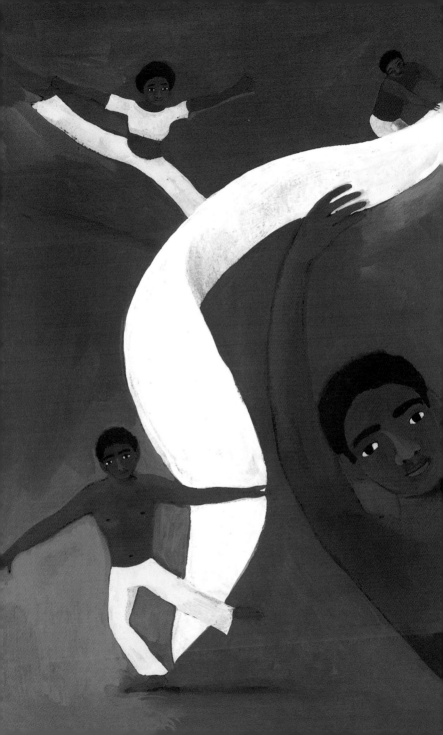

THE ALVIN AILEY DANCE TROUPE

The Alvin Ailey dance troupe has decided to come visit me. I've asked them to perform *Revelations*. Judith Jameson is still dancing, along with the other members of the diminutive company. They are dancing to the spiritual "Wade in the Water." They use a long, thin white cloth, undulating like a ribbon, to make the river of the spiritual come alive. This river is a magnet to my cancer cells, and their conduit out of my body. The dancers are graceful and powerful, statuesque and sure. They move rhythmically through my breast. They are dancing with ecstasy and controlled abandon, and with each undulation of that wide wide ribbon, my cancer cells are ushered farther down the river to flow right out of me.

SPACESHIP

I am tiny and so is this spaceship. It is steel-colored and slender, with two stubby wings sticking out from its back end. On the nose of my spaceship is a gigantic fan with blades that resemble an airplane propeller. These blades are golden, and when they rotate quickly they become a blur of amber light. I am riding my ship through my breast ducts. We are on the prowl for cancer cells. The cells have become close to weightless from the radiation—dry and flat as pancakes. The powerful amber wind from my fan lifts them up and blows them straight out of my breast.

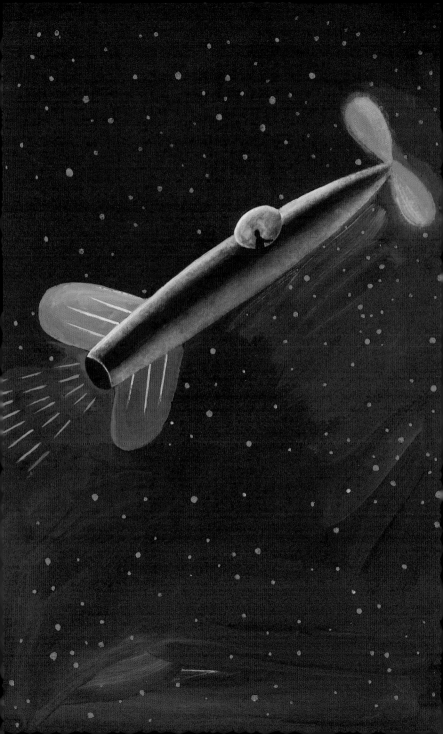

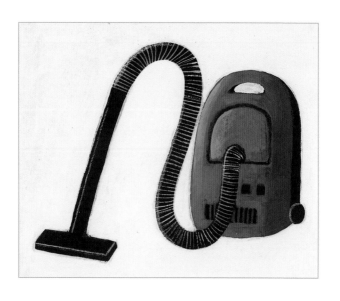

THE VACUUM CLEANER

My heroes have always been firemen. When I was single and toying with the idea of placing a personal ad, it would inevitably say, "Firemen only need apply." In this visualization I have a brigade of small firemen in my breast ducts. They are wearing black rubber suits with yellow boots, and have helmets on their heads. Instead of water hoses, they are wielding giant vacuum cleaners. The suction is powerful, and they methodically go through the tunnels of my breast, sucking out all the cancer cells.

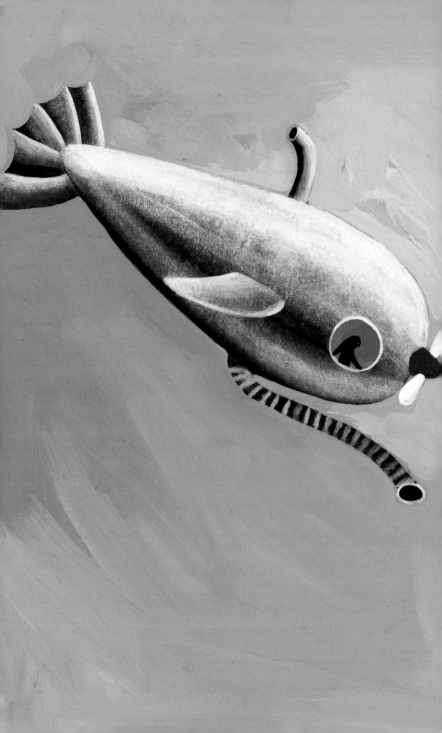

Visualizations
for Treatment:
Chemotherapy

Because chemo takes a much longer time to drip into your body than a round-trip to the radiation table, the visualizations can be done during treatment itself. Being in a comfortable reclining chair is the perfect posture for relaxing into a visualizing state of mind. So get as comfortable as you can, and let your imagination do the rest. When I tried to imagine myself undergoing chemotherapy treatment, this is what I saw:

MINERS WITH SEARCHLIGHTS ON THEIR HATS

The miners are dressed in dark, protective clothing, and each has a headlamp sitting securely on his head. They are perched on little rafts, carried down through the intravenous tubing, into my bloodstream on a healing river of liquid. There are hundreds and hundreds of them, and they all have the high beams of their lanterns turned on, seeking out errant cancer cells. There are so many lamps that my body is lit from within like a field full of fireflies on a warm summer night. The cancer cells disintegrate into harmless dust when they are caught in the powerful beams of the miners' lamps.

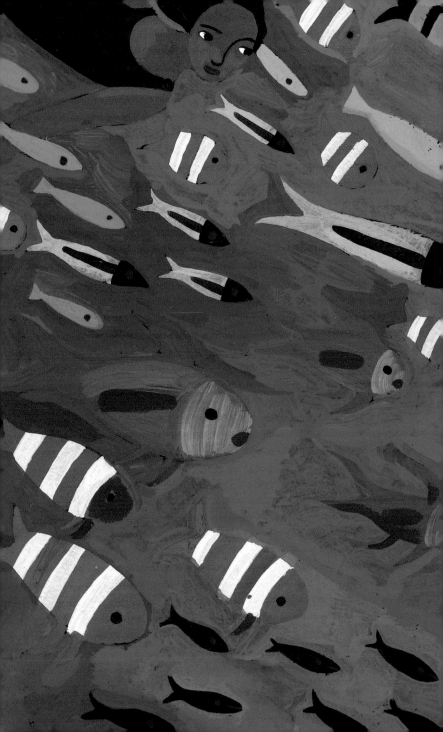

HUNGRY TROPICAL FISH WITH MOUTHS

I am once again diving deep into aquamarine water. I move deeper and deeper down, pulling myself under with powerful strokes of my arms. I have a sense that this water is magical, with healing powers inherent in its makeup. I swim farther and farther away from the surface, and I am surrounded by hundreds of minuscule orange and turquoise tropical fish. Some are yellow and black. I am happy in the company of fish. I realize that they are swimming inside of me as well as outside, and that these fish are hungry! They are microscopic, and can navigate through the narrowest passageways and capillaries of my body. They are hunting cancer cells. When they find them, they snatch them up and gobble them down with gusto. The cancer cells are gone.

THE ACROBATS

My Cirque du Soleil acrobats are Lilliputian. The are *so* small that they each fit inside one drop of the clear liquid dripping down the tubing and into my bloodstream. These teeny-weeny acrobats are dazzling in their brightly colored costumes—a startling visual abundance of red and orange, vermilion and magenta, ochre and gold. The precision and grace of their movements is breathtaking, combining skill and daring to the level of high circus art. They are floating through my bloodstream, twirling and turning somersaults. They are vaulting and diving, doing backflips and pirouettes, a hybrid kind of water ballet. Each acrobat is equipped with scarlet circus netting, spun of the finest silk. They scoop up the cancer cells in nets woven so tightly that not even one molecule can escape, and the cancer cells are carried right out of me.

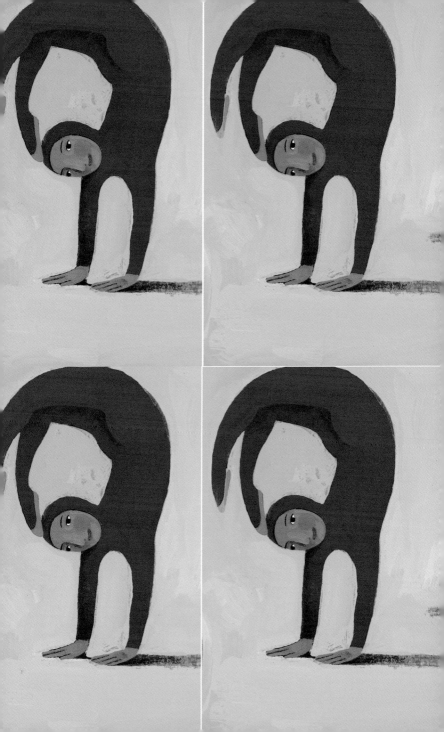

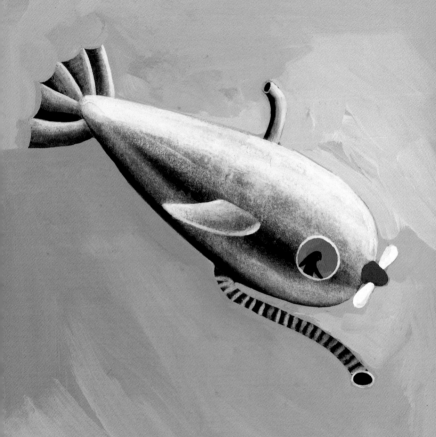

SUBMARINE WITH GIANT SUCTION HOSE

I am aboard a small silver submarine. It is carried along a river of medicine into the waterways and passageways of my body. It can travel through the narrowest of my capillaries. There is a porthole up front, as well as a periscope from which I can peer out and watch for renegade cancer cells. My submarine is equipped with a giant suction hose that protrudes from the underbelly of the ship. When cancer cells are spotted, they are, with tremendous force, sucked into the engine of my submarine, where they are pulverized into harmless dust.

COWGIRLS AT THE RODEO

I am in Elko, Nevada. Three dozen cowgirls, wearing fringed leather shirts and tan leather skirts, are mounted on palominos and roans. They are my private posse—highly skilled cowgirls, on highly trained cow ponies—and they can throw rope with power, accuracy, and aplomb. They are used to roping calves, but for now they have their sights on rambunctious cancer cells. They ride their ponies into the river of chemo, and are carried swiftly in the current throughout my bloodstream. They cover the entire terrain of my body, whooping every time they rope a runaway cancer cell. They are an energetic crew, and the cancer cells don't have a prayer.

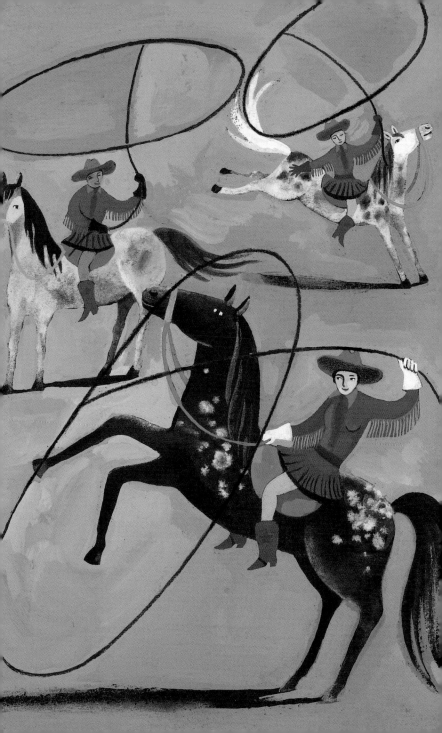

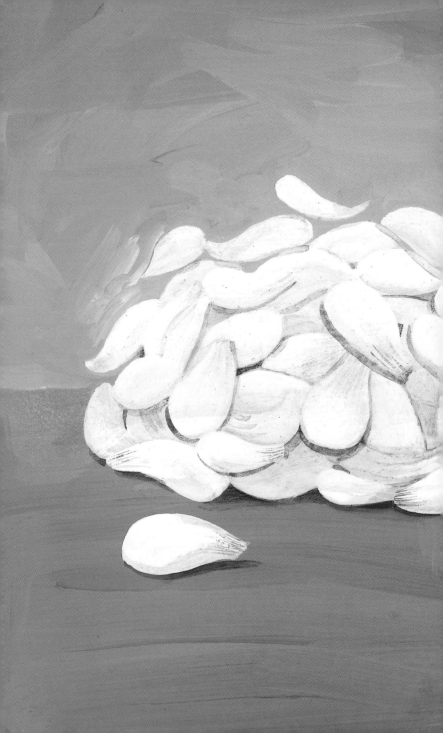

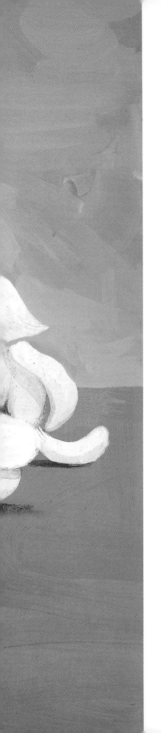

Visualizations *for* Comfort *and* Assistance

The guided imagery tape by Belleruth Naparstek that I was given suggested picking a place to visit in your mind that is safe and beautiful to you. On different days you can visit different places, but each day you can pick only one. Here are a few I visited:

CIRCLE OF FRIENDS

I am up in the Eastern Sierra. I am high above treeline, at twelve thousand feet, and there is green and rust lichen on the rocks under my boots. The snow-covered mountain peaks in front of me are craggy and ancient. The air is crisp and invigorating. It is glorious to be up there. I become aware that I have been joined by a group of my friends. They form a circle around me, and then one of them steps forward, stretching both of her arms out toward me, holding her hands together like a cup, pointing at my breast. The warm healing light of radiation is channeled through those arms and into my breast. I am surrounded by the love and kindness of my friends. I can feel myself healing in the silent, profound beauty of the High Sierra.

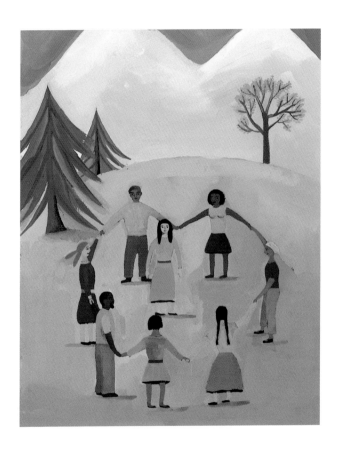

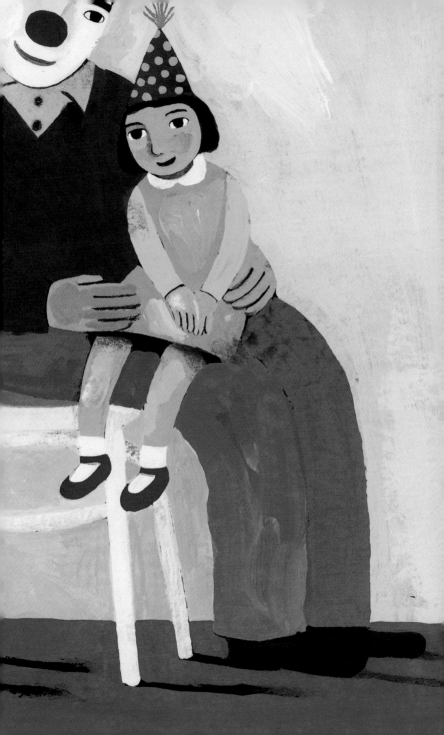

BIRTHDAY PARTY

I am five years old and it is my birthday. Our house is filled with a lot of other five-year-olds, and we are all wearing pointed party hats. My normally buttoned-down father is dressed for the occasion in a clown suit with a red nose. He has decorated his face with white greasepaint. Even at the age of five I know that this is unusual and fairly spectacular. He has done this for *me*. My dad goofs around a bit and we are a very appreciative audience. When the party is over, he sits down in a big white chair and I sit on his lap. His red nose is off, and he holds me quietly in his arms as I absorb this moment into memory. I am safe. I am protected. I am happy. I am loved.

Not all of my visualizations filled me with joy. A few of them left me
with tears streaming down my cheeks. At first I worried about this.
Aren't I supposed to be making myself feel better? But I realized that
the sadness I was experiencing was part of the process I was going
through, and it was healthier for me to actually let it run through
me than to ignore it or pretend it wasn't there.

So I made welcome the sadness that at times came flooding through.
And took comfort as well in what I imagined. If this happens to you,
my advice is to let it wash through you. You need to feel sad. This is
what that sadness looked liked for me:

MA-MA

I want so much to go to someplace safe. I am longing for comfort. I close my eyes and find myself snuggled deeply in my mother's arms. The last time I can remember actually being in this position was when my mother was dying of cancer. I had crawled into bed with her and was wrapped up softly in her arms. This image hurt a lot. But I stayed there—crying and hugging her in my mind—soaking her up. When I finished the visualization I was still very sad. Maybe I'm doing this wrong, I thought. I'm not supposed to make myself feel worse. Then it happened a second time. This time my mom was the person who stepped forward out of my circle of friends to guide me through the radiation. Tears were running down my face as I stayed in the circle and watched her beautiful face. I felt her helping administer my treatment. I realized what a gift it was that I could conjure her at all—that she had metaphorically crossed a great distance in order to be with me and lend me comfort. And comfort was what I felt.

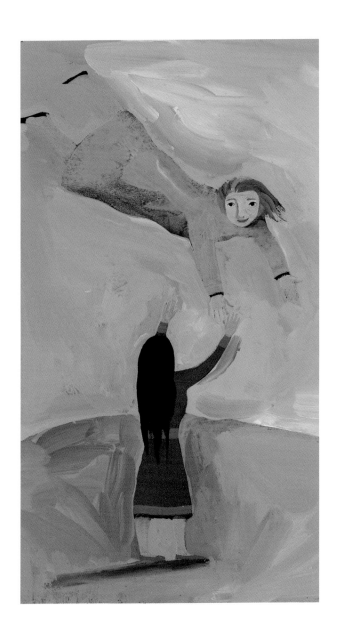

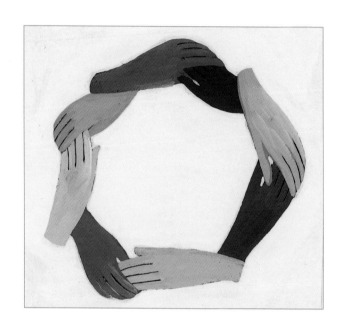

DEATH VALLEY

This is not as ominous as it sounds. I am in an amber canyon in Death Valley, California. There are rock formations on either side of me, and the sky is a rich desert blue. The sand underfoot is amber colored too. The entire canyon glows in the sunlight. Again I find myself in the center of a circle of friends. This time they have their arms around one another's shoulders and they stand so close to me that all of us are touching. No one says a word. I just soak up their warmth and their love for me. My gratitude is enormous. I know I am being healed.

MA-MA, PART TWO

After the tearful reunions, I was able to visualize my mother in a different way. Experiencing her deep and unconditional love for me became a cornerstone of my practice. I close my eyes and in a relaxed state I can literally feel the sweetness and strength of her love for me. The gentleness of her nature and the depth of her love are sustenance to me. I let that pure energy flow like a river into my veins, filling me up with safety and joy. For me, this gift of energizing love comes from my mother. For you, it might come from a beloved grandparent, a child, or a pet. The source doesn't matter. It is an infusion that sustains, lifting me up, making me want to do the Happy Dance.

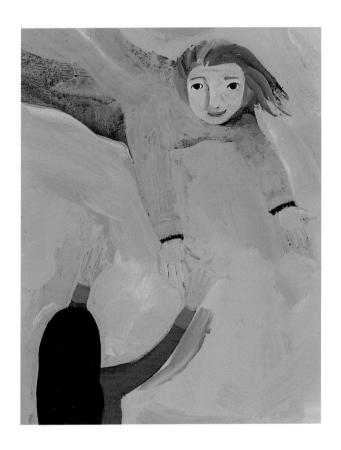

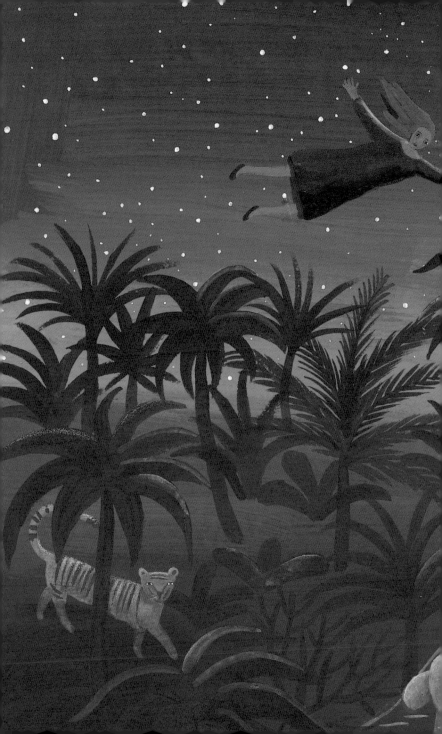

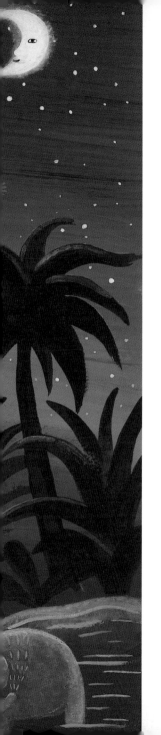

Visualizations
for Energy

*When I started radiation therapy I was
told that fatigue would likely be one of
the side effects I would experience. It is
my understanding that chemotherapy is
often more exhausting than radiation.
I told myself that if fatigue came I would
try to honor it, but at the same time I
wanted to try to mine sources of energy
deep within myself. This is what I imagined:*

THE HAPPY DANCE

I am in a field out in Carmel Valley, where Robert Louis Stevenson once had a cabin. The field is covered with lupine and poppies. It has high green and wheat-colored grass, and is a virtual sea of purple and orange flowers. There is an enormous oak tree in the center of this field, and at first I think I will go sit down and rest against its trunk—drawing in its strength by simply sitting there. But then I surprise myself. Much to my astonishment I am doing somersaults in the flowers. I am leaping high in the air like Nureyev, and doing backflips like my acrobats. SIT DOWN!!!!! I scold myself, Owen Meany–style. YOU'RE SUPPOSED TO BE RESTING! But I ignore my more pedantic self, and continue to leap and cavort in the air, dancing and laughing myself silly. I have come to this field, apparently, to celebrate the power of joy.

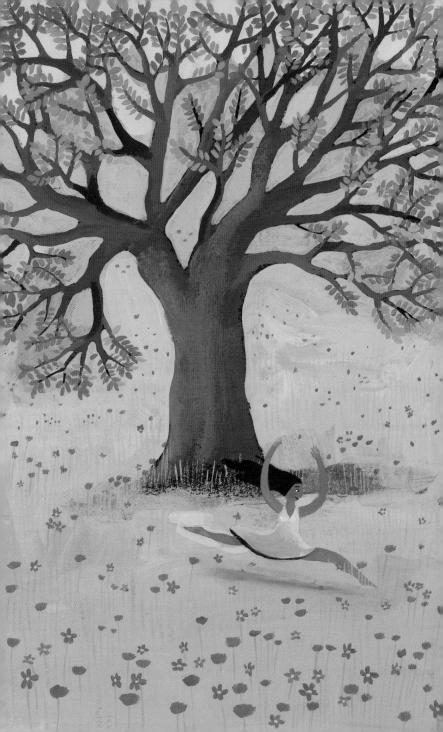

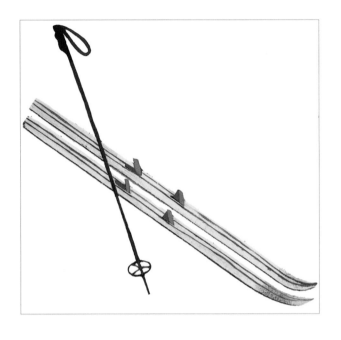

SKIING

I am not, in real life, much of a skier. I am anything but intrepid on the slopes. Frankly, the velocity of downhill skiing scares the wits out of me. But in this visualization I am fearless. I am perched atop a very high peak in the Rocky Mountains. The air is arctic and I can see my breath every time I exhale. The white snow is everywhere. I'm wearing sunglasses because it is so bright, and a fetching purple ski suit. The sky is mountain blue. I take a deep breath and go careening down a very steep slope. I am moving like a bullet, gathering more speed every second. I am not afraid. All I feel is the thrill of motion as the white world whips by me in a blur and I fly.

CANYON DE CHELLY

I am in the Arizona desert with my friend Ki. We are at Canyon de Chelly, a red-rock canyon tucked into the northeastern corner of the state. New Mexico is just across the border. We are in a field, in a flat section of the canyon that stretches for miles. We are riding Navaho horses. I am on a chestnut gelding, and he quickly moves from a spirited canter to a no-nonsense gallop and then before I know it into a flat-out, full-blown, breathtaking run. I am leaning forward in the saddle and have my arms wound tightly around his neck. He smells warm and oatey, his coat sparkles in the golden sunlight, and we are flying! We are running so fast we seem to lift off the ground entirely, and soar with unbridled energy through the clear desert air. I look to my left, and my friend on her pinto is flying right alongside me, as flushed with excitement as I am.

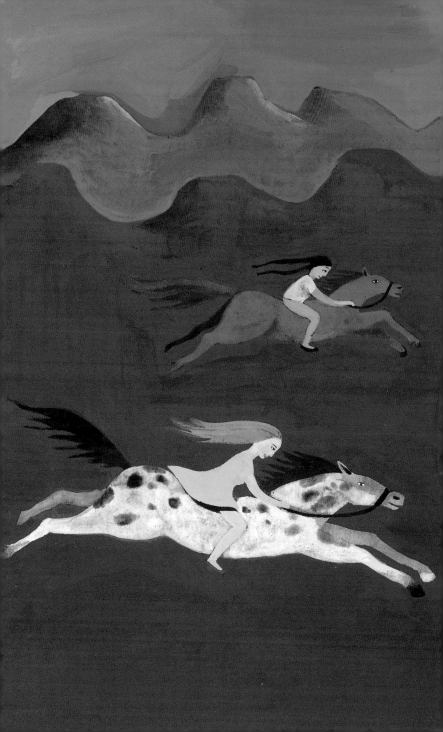

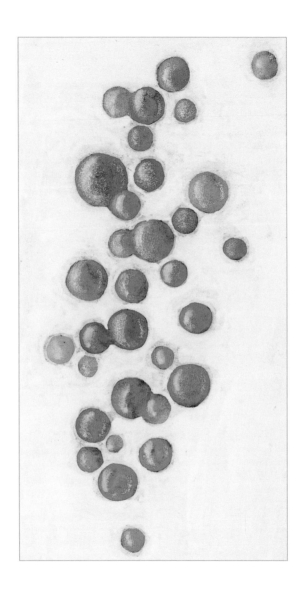

THE UNDERWATER SPRING

Once again I am diving underwater, but the water is dark and cool. I can't see very much at all, but that doesn't concern me. I just keep pulling myself deeper and deeper under. Breathing is not a problem. I can breathe in the water. I am like a fish, sounding. I have no desire to stop. So down and down and down I swim, the world above me disappearing entirely. Water is the only element I know. Finally I reach an underwater shelf at the bottom of the lake or ocean I am in. A cool, clear spring of water is bubbling upward like a Jacuzzi. It is so refreshing. I just hover there, and let the spring send crystal clear energy right into my veins. I am alive with this energy. Slowly I swim back up to the surface feeling refreshed and ready to rock.

FLYING

I close my eyes and I am airborne in a midnight blue sky. I am stretched out on my belly; just like a childhood dream, my arms are straight out on either side of my head and I am flying. The air is cool and I feel invigorated. There is a yellow crescent moon, straight out of a children's book. Stars are silver and shaped like, well, stars. I see the earth below me. It is silent where I am. I can almost hear the Milky Way. I glide over houses where everyone is fast asleep. I glide over gardens and cats out on the prowl. I fly over jungles where tigers are hunting, and elephants are frolicking in muddy water, over monasteries where novices are meditating, over three rock climbers who are sleeping in hammocks on the face of El Capitan! I am alone but I'm not at all frightened. It is exhilarating to be out here in the night. And when my visualization is over, I stay filled with the energy of that weightless velocity.

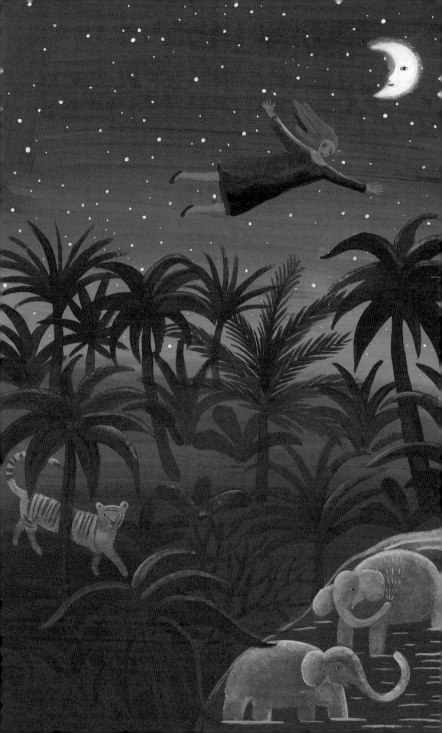

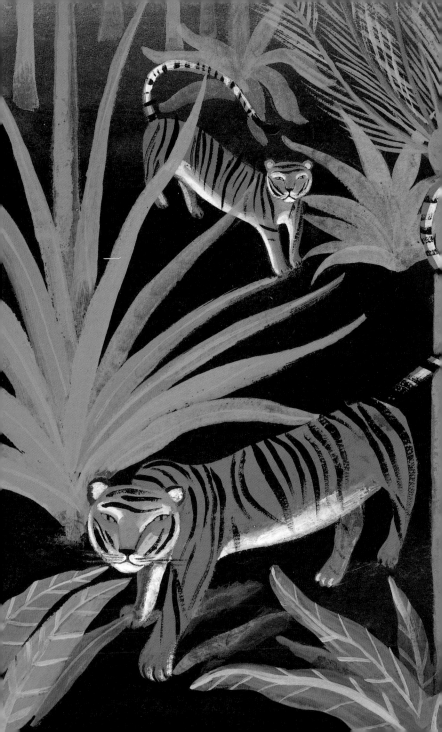

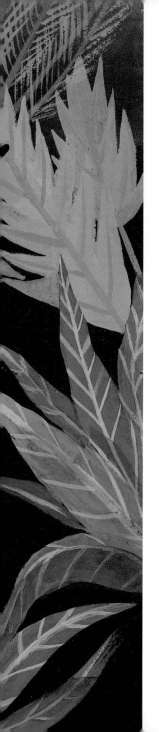

Visualizations *to* Overcome Fear

During the course of my treatment, I felt frightened a few times. Odd as it may seem, it wasn't about the cancer except once, when I started worrying about its reappearing after my treatment was over. But more often, old fears came to visit, fears that have been my companions time and time again. I realized one day that I could use visualization and even the radiation to help me vaporize these fears—to send them out into the universe and away from me. This is what I imagined:

RADIANT HEAT

It is so simple. I give myself the morning off as far as visualizing my cancer cells being baked into nothingness. Instead, I focus that radiant beam on a very old fear that has shadowed me for as long as I can remember. I let the full, magnificent power of the radiant light bear down on this fear as I breathe slowly and rhythmically, watching my fear dissolve into carbon dioxide that I exhale away.

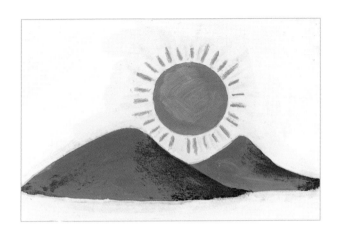

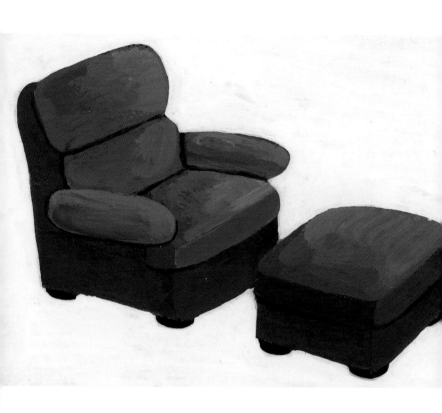

ALCHEMY

Once again, this visualization takes a time-out from focusing on treatment to pulverize cancer cells and this time turns the power of chemotherapy on fear itself. Fear is a palpable emotion. Its presence makes my heart beat faster and my breath short. I am lying comfortably on a lounge chair. The drip is about to begin. I visualize the powerful liquid medicine entering my bloodstream and seeking out my fear. The medicine can sniff it, and therefore it can dissolve it. I relax and smile at the beauty of this.

HELIUM BALLOONS

I am inside my own bloodstream. I have a little canister with me that resembles an oxygen tank. But it has my fear inside it instead, and I fill up hundreds of balloons with this fear. Ruby red, bright orange, Crayola crayon yellow. The balloons fill up and my fear, it turns out, is as light as helium. They rise in a flock and I exhale them through my nose. I take a deep breath and remind myself that my fear has floated away. I have the power to make it so.

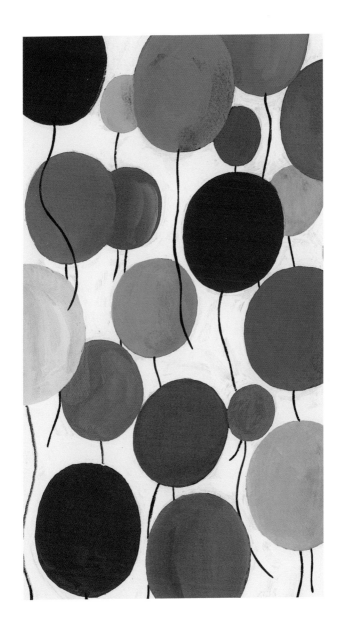

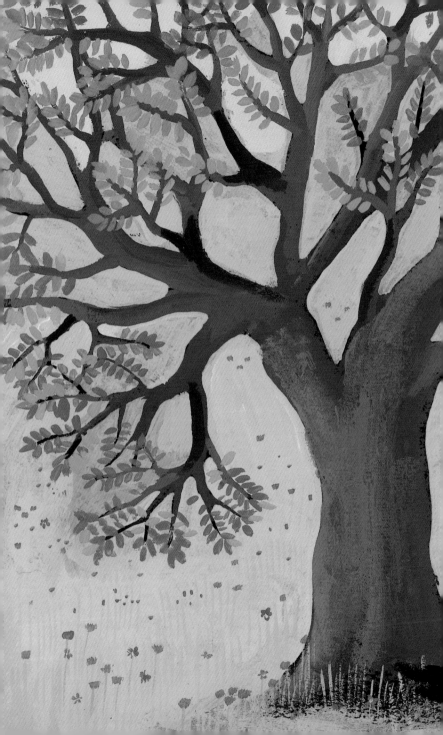

MY FIELD OF LUPINE

I am frightened, so I find myself returning to a place I know is safe. It is my field in Carmel Valley, which is awash in purple lupine and orange California poppies. The smell of the lupine is intensely sweet. It is *such* a beautiful field. There is a giant oak, and I sit myself down on the soft grass beneath it and wait. Eventually I see a familiar and beloved figure approaching. It is my mother, and she glides up to me, sits down on the ground, and takes both of my hands in her own. She knows that I am frightened. She tells me over and over again that the world is full of bounty, and that, already inside of me I have everything I need to feel safe and happy, everything I need to be healthy and unafraid. I believe her when she tells me this. I stand up and gather a bouquet of lupine for her. I know that I will be able to call up her words of assurance and comfort the next time I feel anxious or afraid, wherever I might be.

Visualizations
for Healing

*I can't actually imagine what my breast
tissue has had to endure throughout the
course of three surgeries, two needle
localizations, and thirty-three exposures
to radiation. Even with my beloved beach
umbrellas, I have to assume that the tissue
has experienced trauma and dehydration.
I decide to visualize that tissue healing
and regenerating. This is what I see:*

ROSEWATER AND HONEY

For this visualization I am in my garden. This place brings me joy. Once there, I sit down amidst the flowers and can see that my breast tissue is a beautiful shade of peach. I see the tissue bathed in a mixture of glycerin and rosewater with a touch of honey. It has grown plump and soft, moist and resilient. I stand and shake loose the velvety petals of a dozen white peonies. I sprinkle them, in a fragrant blanket, over my breast. I picture my tissue snuggling down under this blanket to mend.

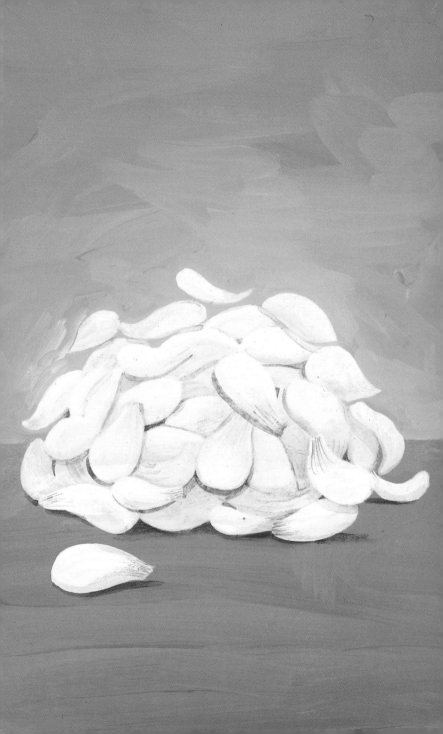

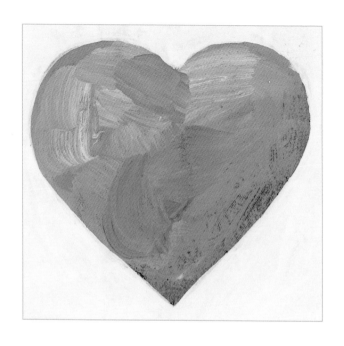

MY PEACH-COLORED THYMUS GLAND

Although I've always had my thymus gland with me, tucked safely under my breastbone, I'd never paid any mind to it before being diagnosed with breast cancer. Only then did I discover its importance in keeping me healthy. A tiny bit of science, for those as oblivious as I was about its function: the thymus gland is central to the functioning of our immune system. Half of the white blood cells that we produce head into our bloodstream, and half of them are cycled through the thymus, where they morph into T lymphocytes. These little champions stimulate the growth and production of antibodies by other lymphocytes, stimulate the growth and production of phagocytes, whose job is to surround and neutralize viruses and bacteria, and, very importantly, they can detect and destroy abnormal tissue. So I learned to love my thymus gland, and the microscopic gladiators it produces on my behalf.

In this visualization I picture my thymus beneath my breastbone. In my mind's eye it is heart shaped and peach-colored. It is plump and moist. It is glowing with health and energy. It is a busy gland, fat and sassy, and if it could wink at me it would—letting me know that it is fit as a fiddle and keeping me well stocked with my all-important T cells.

THE BEACH

I imagine myself on a beach in the early summer. The ocean is calm, with gentle waves lapping along the shore. I am alone on a long stretch of white sand that goes on for miles, as far as my eye can see. It is flawless. I feel a deep sense of contentment when I look out to the horizon and see the perfection of this uninterrupted stretch of warm, white sand. The resonance and comfort is deep within me. I intuitively know that the cancer cells are gone from my body—melted away and vanished. I breathe deeply and feel myself quietly glowing with health.

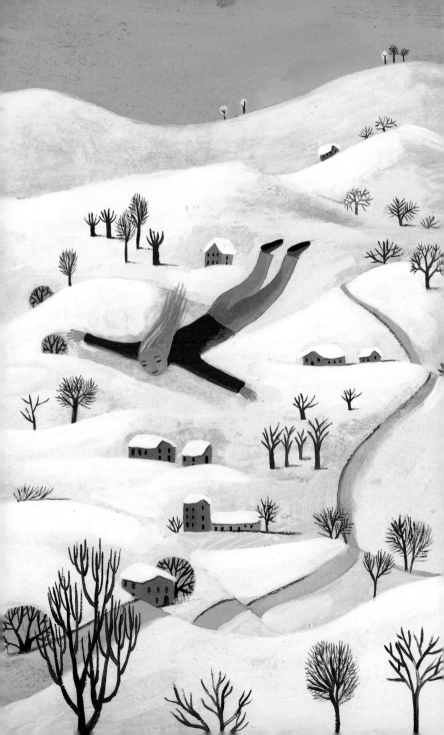

SNOW

This image came to me the day after my treatment ended. It was less of a visualization than a realization that I felt tremendously drawn to the image of vast fields covered in snow. It is winter here in the Hudson Valley, and snow is, for the time being, our element. I feel a deep sense of peace when I gaze out on unblemished fields of snow, stretching to the horizon as far as I can see. The resonance I feel is on a cellular level. I instinctively know that the cancer cells are gone from my body, that the tissue is as clean and pure as the snow that surrounds me. I close my eyes and luxuriate in this feeling of absolute health. In my visualization I am flying over a great field of snow. It blankets the ground for acres, and I slowly survey all of it from above, seeing it is flawless. I hold this quiet realization inside of me. I am healed.

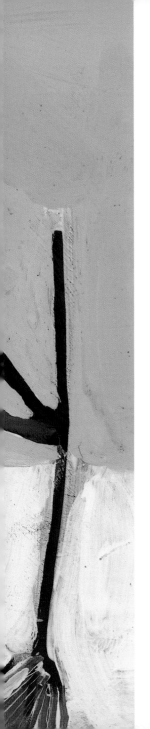

Visualizations *for* Continuing Health

The day my treatment was over was an extremely emotional one for me. Although I only had one or two crying sessions of deluge proportions from the time I was diagnosed through my entire treatment, the floodgates opened while I was still at the hospital, trying to thank my astonishing team of caregivers. I could barely speak. I was so moved by their kindness, generosity, and concern for me. Once I left the hospital I realized that the medical phase of treating my cancer was pretty much over, except for follow-up mammograms and visits with my physicians . I wanted to be able to move forward and protect and nurture my new-found health. While deeply relaxed, I can assure myself that I have everything within me that I need to be happy and stay healthy. Visualizations will allow me to do just that.

CIRQUE DU SOLEIL ACROBATS REDUX

Fortunately for me, my Cirque du Soleil acrobats do not have to move on to another city now that my treatment is over. They can stay with me indefinitely, and I can equip them with magnifying glasses and deep crimson circus nets made of silk. They are on constant patrol all over my body, circulating through my breast ducts and bloodstream and lymphatic system. They are vigilant, inspecting my interior terrain for hibernating cancer cells. They watch out for me while I am awake, and while I sleep. And if they *do* find any errant cancer cells lurking, they will sweep them up in their nets and usher them to the nearest exit.

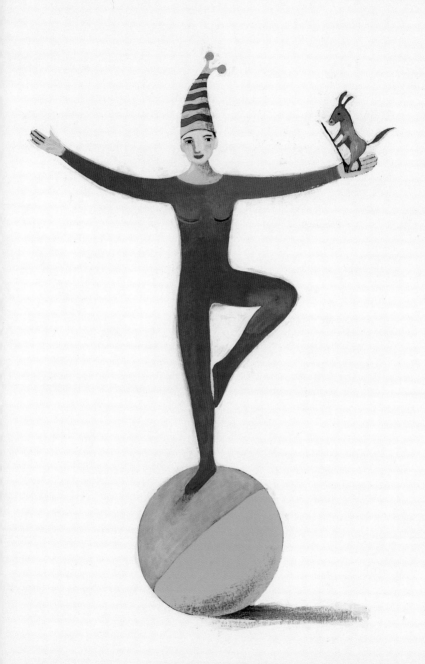

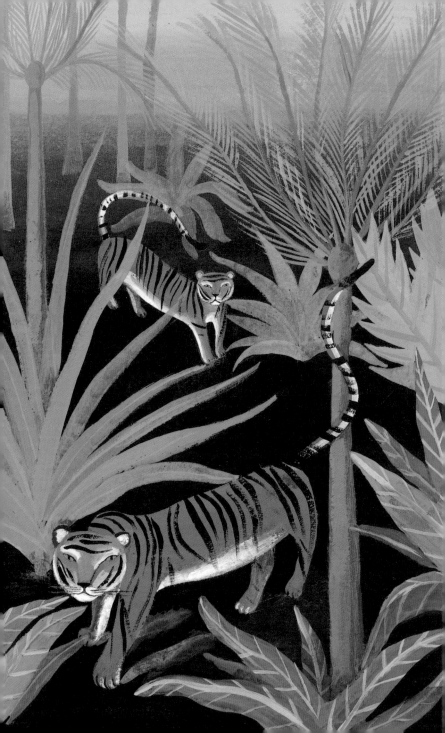

MY BENGAL TIGERS

They are magnificent adult male tigers: orange and black and white. Their power and authority are palpable. I can see their muscles ripple as they swing their massive shoulders and prowl throughout my body. They are hunting. They are seeking out any cancer cells that are foolish enough to try to take up residence in the territory of my body. The tigers are fearsome, but produce only awe and gratitude in me. I know they are constantly alert, and their hunting comes from a deep, primal place. They are keeping me safe.

ENERGY FORCE

I relax deeply, using a hypnotic technique that has me climb down three sets of mental stairs to a place I chose in Maine that offers me quiet, joyful tranquility. I'm sitting on a large boulder at water's edge. The sun has already set, and light is quickly fading, leaving the sky gradations of soft red to deepening twilight blue. The water is mirror calm, and close to black in color. I concentrate, and can feel a powerful force field emanating from deep within me. It is a force that originates on an atomic level, and it protects each and every one of my cells from harm. The force exists as a kind of antimagnet, to repel any cancer cells from forming or taking root inside of me. As I breathe quietly, and stay gently focused, I am aware of it being ever present in my body.

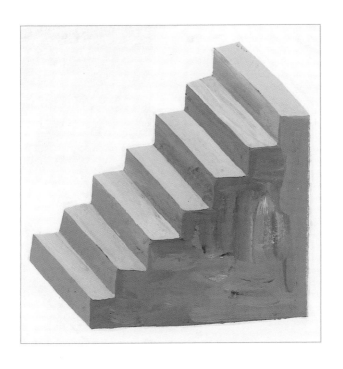

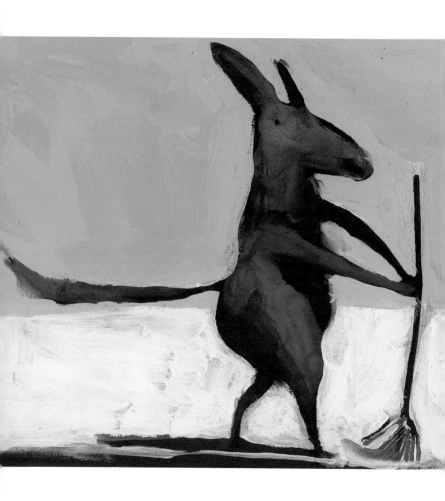

THE LONE SWEEPER

I have been befriended by a blue donkey with a broom. He walks on his hind legs, and he is entirely devoted to sweeping my breast ducts clean. He hardly ever sleeps. His broom is his passion, and like Sam the Lion's son Billy in Peter Bogdanovich's *The Last Picture Show,* he is happy when he is sweeping. He is my constant companion, ever vigilant with his broom, making sure my breast ducts remain forever clear of marauding cancer cells.

SEA OF TRANQUILITY

*One benefit of experiencing cancer was that the world slowed down
for me. Days of hectic activity and stressful overload came to an
abrupt halt when my focus was shifted to mending from surgery and
then the daily practice of radiation therapy. I know that an ancillary
benefit of the visualizations was my embracing this slower pace.
I started to breathe more deeply and shift my priorities a bit. "Does
this really matter enough for me to twist my shorts in a knot over
it?" Often my answer to myself is "No." Holding on to this more
tranquil state of mind has become a way to provide comfort to
myself. This is what I see:*

I am sitting in the lotus position, a middle-aged baby Buddha.
I am sitting on a cloud straight out of a children's book, floating
in a powder blue sky. I breathe in and out quietly, and feel an
overwhelming sense of gratitude to be here on this planet, at
this moment in time, with the friends and family that I have
and the gift of stillness that I have been given. My cloud floats
over the turquoise of an ocean. The world is silent for a
moment, and I feel blessed to be alive.

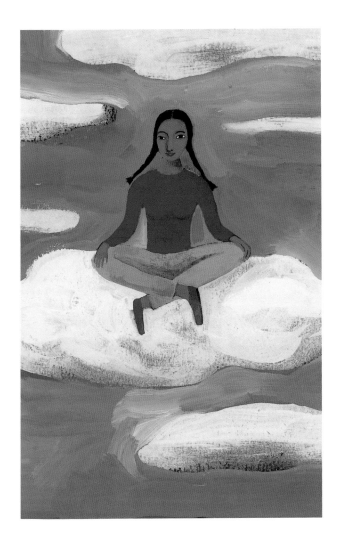

I always wondered whether, if I ever wrote a book, I would be one of those people who thanks a cast of thousands. The answer appears to be yes.

For their generosity of spirit, and for the love and kindness they showed me while I was deep within the cancer journey, I would like to thank the following people: Dr. Emily Sonnenblick, for her keen eyesight and gentle manner. Dr. Alexander Swistel, for his warmth, humanity, and remarkable skill as a surgeon: you are the Stradivarius of surgeons. Pat Burbridge, who opened the magical door of visualizations for me. Rob Wallin and the men and women of the Dyson Cancer Center at the Vassar Brothers Medical Center in Poughkeepsie, who were unfailingly kind, and who made my daily treatments as close to joyful as is humanly possible. Dr. Michael Kauff for his wise counsel. Dr. Edward Faranghi, who patiently answered my many questions.

My friends and family have offered no less than astonishing love and support. They raised my spirits, always listened, and helped me to feel safe. Boundless gratitude goes to Steven and Pauline Burton, Caroline Herter, Chris Lloreda, Tom Stanley, Mary Shapiro, Macduff Everton, Mary Heebner, Nell Campbell, Ann Patty, Ann Smith, Marianne Brogan, Barb Parmet, Lena Tabori, Jeff Briley, Maria Marewski, Linda and Jim Mulvey and the three little Mulveys, M Mark for her friendship and for the remarkable gift of her editing pencil, Thérèse Burke, Ronnie Rowes, Craig Krull, Joost Elffers, Leonard and Joan Berger, Nancy and Michael Horowitz, Arla and David Coffey, Abel Shafer, Susan and Arnold Wechsler, Polly Hahn, Donna Zulch, the extraordinary staff at IXL Health Club, and of course to my beloved Bubba: you are my greatest gift. Heartfelt thanks to Simona Mulazzani whose beautiful illustrations bring me so much joy, and to Daniele Melani and Gail Gaynin.

Lastly, I was blessed to find a loving, nurturing, and extremely enthusiastic home for this project at Harmony Books, and I particularly want to express my gratitude to Kim Kanner Meisner, Shaye Areheart, Philip Patrick, and Felix Gregorio.

God bless you all.

Selected Reading and Listening

Breast Cancer: Beyond Convention. Edited by Mary Tagliaferri, M.D., L.Ac.; Issac Cohen, O.M., L.Ac.; and Debu Tripathy, M.D. New York: Atria Books, 2002.

Dr. Susan Love's Breast Book, 3rd ed. Susan M. Love, M.D., with Karen Lindsey. Massachusetts: Perseus Publishing, 2000.
www.susanlove.com

Self-Hypnotism: The Technique and Its Use in Daily Living. Leslie M. LeCron. New York: Signet Books, 1989.

Staying Well with Guided Imagery. Belleruth Naparstek. New York: Warner Books, 1995.

Relaxation and Guided Imagery for People Undergoing Radiation Therapy. Belleruth Naparstek. Ohio: Image Paths, Inc., 1999.
www.healthjourneys.com

A Guided Imagery Tape for People Undergoing Chemotherapy. Belleruth Naparstek. Ohio: Image Paths, Inc., 1991.
www.healthjourneys.com

Wendy Burton has worked in the publishing industry for over twenty-seven years, both in Northern California and in New York City. She is a photographer, book designer, and freelance literary agent specializing in visual books. She lives in Red Hook, New York, with her husband, Jeff Brouws. *Joy Is a Plum Colored Acrobat* is her first book.